Contents

What is a Kamado Grill?

A kamado grill, to put it simply, is similar to the rounded, kettle shaped charcoal grill we all grew up with. Whereas standard charcoal grills are shaped like a dome and made of metal, Kamado Grills are typically oval shaped and look much like a large urn or even an egg. This design actually originated in Japan some 3,000 years ago when people first used Kamados to cook rice and then later installed a cooking grid for grilling and roasting meats.

History of the Kamado

Early clay ovens appeared in China about 3,000 years ago. (The Chinese, as you may recall, also developed the fire-hardened clay we now call ceramics, as well as porcelain coatings.) Around

300 BC, this technology was exported to Japan, and the ceramic ovens were dubbed kamados, or "stoves."

How did the kamado come to the States? After World War II, thousands of Westerners stationed in Japan saw these wonderful cookers for the first time. Returning home, many brought kamados back, and some even started importing and selling them. One such entrepreneur was Ed Fisher, who sensed there might be an interest in these ceramic charcoal burners back in the USA. In 1974, he opened a store in Atlanta, and the Big Green Egg was born. Big Green Egg is now the most popular brand of kamado in the world, with legions of devotees who affectionately call themselves Eggheads.

But the Big Green Egg isn't the only kamado out there. You now have a wide range of choices in all different sizes, shapes, and colors.

Advantages of Oval-Shaped Kamados and Problems of Round Kamados

We are strong believers in the two-zone system for grilling. The concept is to place the coals on one side of the grill and leave the other side without coals. On a gas grill, you turn on the burners on one side, but not on the other. With two zones, you can move food from very hot, direct radiant infrared heat to mild, indirect convection heat, quickly and easily.

Oval-shaped kamados, like those made by Primo and Komodo Kamado, can easily be set up for two-zone cooking, but round kamados cannot.

The oval shape enables more separation from side to side, while heat in the round models tends to even out rather quickly. Most round-kamado aficionados concede that their best way of creating different heat zones is by moving foods closer to or farther from the fire. This is done with various deflectors and rack systems that can be costly and awkward to manipulate.

Can You Grill on a Kamado?

Kamados can get mighty hot. We cranked a Big Green Egg until a column of fire shot out the top, and it was like a blast furnace inside. That's great for searing the snot out of thin meats, like skirt steak, that you just want to cook hot and fast, but (as mentioned above) once kamados get hot, they take forever to cool down. Along with the difficulty of creating a two-zone setup, this is why we believe most kamados function better as smokers and ovens than as grills.

If you really want to take your grilling skills to the highest level, then you need to master two-zone cooking and get a charcoal grill in addition to the kamado, or select a kamado that can do two-zone cooking.

Is It Okay to Use Regular Charcoal Briquettes?

Many kamado manufacturers recommend or even dictate that you use more expensive lump charcoal rather than briquettes. They argue that briquettes produce more ash than lump, and the ash can block airflow as it builds up over long cooks. Most kamado manufacturers also sell private-label lump charcoal, so they just might have a conflict of interest. Generally, we recommend using Kingsford Original Briquets in charcoal burners, because they're affordable, consistent, and readily available. Lump charcoal, especially the bargain-basement varieties, can be inconsistent. We've seen bags that were half pulverized charcoal dust and half large chunks of construction material. It's not unusual to find metal and plastic debris mixed in. Nonetheless, I personally prefer high-quality lump in a kamado over briquettes, because it's lighter and easier to stir around at the bottom of the deep firebox, while briquettes tend to get compacted.

Firing Up a Kamado

Do not use lighter fluid to start your charcoal in any ceramic cooker; that stuff can get into the porous interior, which is bad news. Instead, it's best to always use a chimney, electric starter, or firestarter.

Here's a trick we learned from Dennis Linkletter of Komodo Kamado: Fill the charcoal basket, bury one Weber paraffin firestarter cube in the pile of charcoal, and light it. It will ignite about five briquettes immediately around it. They will burn slowly, producing very little heat, and the combustion will spread gradually to unlit coals. When shooting for low-and-slow smoking temps of 225°F (105°C), once you get a fist-sized cluster of briquettes glowing, it's already time to shut down both the lower intake damper and upper exhaust damper to let just a small amount of air in and out. The smart move is to let your kamado slowly come up to the desired temp and stabilize, rather than risk overshooting your mark.

Easy as it is to maintain temps over a long period in these stable cookers, some like to go a step further and use thermostatic temperature controllers, like the popular BBQ Guru, which control cooking temperature by regulating a small fan affixed to the air intake damper. These gizmos enable you to run a kamado for days at low-and-slow smoking temps, with no babysitting.

What are the Benefits of a Kamado Grill?

There are several ways Kamado Grills can benefit the backyard griller who is looking to enhance their outdoor cooking experience:

Versatility

Kamado Grills are exceptional for grilling, smoking, baking, BBQ, and roasting. This versatility allows the outdoor cook many unique options in one grill.

Feel like making a true wood fired pizza ? Because of its design, kamado grills make exceptional pizza ovens since they are extremely efficient at insulating and circulating heat throughout the grill. This results in a crispy bottom crust while perfectly melting the top layer of cheese.

And don't forget about the classics either. Steaks, ribs, burgers, the Kamado can cook them all with that classic lump charcoal flavor. S

Flavor

Kamado Grills use wood lump charcoal which results in a tasty smoke and charcoal flavor that is classically associated with grilling.

Ceramic charcoal grills also do a tremendous job at retaining the moisture of whatever you are cooking. Since air is locked tightly, your meat remains more tender and juicier than it would on a regular charcoal grill

Steady Temperatures

Since Kamado Grills are so well insulated, temperatures hold relatively steady for longer periods of time compared to a traditional charcoal grill. There is a learning curve to controlling temperatures as you will need to play around with the dampers to balance the intake and outflow of air.

In short:

More air = more heat, less air = less heat.

Longevity

As long as you treat your Kamado with care (and don't drop it from a height where it can crack), it should last a very long time.

Maintenance is Simple

Cleaning and maintaining a Kamado Grill is a breeze. Simply clean your grates and gently brush out the bottom. The ceramic is self-cleaning so do not use a wire brush as they can damage the surface.

A Great Grill for the Winter

Because Kamados are constructed to have such effective insulation, cold temperatures do not have the same effect on internal temperatures as it does on other grills. You may have to use more fuel to bring your grill up to its desired temperature, but once it reaches that temp, it will hold much better than a standard charcoal or propane grill.

Top Kamado Grill

But first, a cooker. Should you go for the Green Egg or look for another brand? Here are my top kamado cookers for your consideration.

Uncrackable: Char-Griller Akorn Kamado Grill

The Akorn is a double-walled, insulated steel egg that is much lighter and in some ways more durable than the popular Big Green Egg—and it's less than half the price. Char-Griller has mostly been known over the years for inexpensive grills, and, until now, you pretty much got what you paid for. But this design and Char-Griller's manufacturing process may be a match made in heaven. This cooker performs fairly close to traditional kamados at a fraction of the cost. Don't expect the Akorn to last forever, but if you're curious about kamados and you've been waiting for the right time and price, this could be it.

Cooking Area: 302 square inches (about 14 burgers)

All Hands on Deck: Char-Broil Kamander Charcoal Grill

Char-Broil's Kamander Charcoal Grill, despite the name, is actually a kamado (the Kamander is a kamado—get it?). In keeping with Char-Broil's aim of removing consumer pain points, the Kamander has a list price of just $349.99—far less than a basic Big Green Egg with a stand, which runs about $1,000. That makes it one of the lowest-cost kamados on the market, potentially lifting the biggest barrier many consumers have to buying one of these cookers.

The Kamander is heavier and sturdier than the cheaper Akorn and features a unique airflow design, with the air intake vent at cooking-grate level rather than on the bottom of the cooker (saving you the annoyance of having to bend over to adjust the intake damper). The large removable ash pan makes dumping ashes easy, and the ring of air intake holes around it aids in uniform air circulation.

Of course, a few corners have been cut to achieve the Kamander's wallet-friendliness, but it delivers a solid kamado cooking experience at a price point way below that of most other brands.

Cooking Area: 327 square inches (about 16 burgers)

Self-Starter: Vision Professional S-Series Kamado

Vision's Professional S-Series kamado has some unique and interesting features not found on other ceramic cookers. The bottom dampers are part of a slide-out ash drawer, which also has a slot for the included electric starter. And you gotta love the stainless steel two-level grates: The top grate is hinged for easy access to the lower level, which is also hinged for adding wood and tending to charcoal. This nice package deal includes a solid, powder-coated stand on four casters, with fold-down wood side shelves and a cover.

Vision's goal is to make use easier—easier start-up, easier ash removal. To this end, Vision created an optional Quickchange Gas Insert that may be swapped in for the slide-out ash drawer, turning the S-Series from a kamado to a gas grill when you want to grill up a quick weeknight dinner. Quickchange is a slide-out, 25,000-BTU stainless steel burner that includes a heat exchanger and Vision's round Lava Stone diffuser and stainless steel bracket.

Cooking Area: 302 square inches (about 14 burgers)

Rule the Backyard Roost: Big Green Egg Large Ceramic Cooker

Many view the Big Green Egg as the Weber of kamados. Big Green Egg popularized kamado cookers in the US, and it's often viewed as the industry standard. In fact, some competitors design their kamados to work with Big Green Egg accessories. Big Green Eggs are available in seven models in progressively larger diameters, from 10 inches to 29 inches, but this "Large Egg" (18 inches in diameter) is the most popular size—big enough for a 20-pound turkey. The BGE design is simple and built to last, with a limited lifetime warranty. They're manufactured in Mexico.

When you buy an Egg, you start with just the ceramic oven, and everything else is à la carte. By the time you add a few basics, like a stand and diffuser plate, the cost has gone up significantly. Eggs are not sold on the internet, but they have a lot of dealers coast to coast, so you shouldn't have much trouble getting your hands on one.

Cooking Area: 262 square inches (about 12 burgers)

Super Bowl of 'Cue: Grill Dome Infinity Series (Large)

Grill Domes are known for heavy construction, with top-quality 304-grade stainless steel, excellent heat retention, and beautiful enamel finishes. The ceramic was developed by Grill Dome founder Tarsem Kohli in Atlanta. Called Terapex, it's more durable than traditional ceramic, Grill Dome claims, and can withstand much higher temperatures. Instead of a ceramic-glaze finish, the six colors available come in baked-on enamel. The company believes these finishes help mitigate crazing, the tiny cracks that can form across the exteriors of glazed kamados. Either way, they sure are pretty.

Cooking Area: 254 square inches (about 12 burgers)

Two-Zone Kamado: Primo Oval JR

We'll go ahead and say it: We like these cookers better than the popular Big Green Egg. As mentioned above, kamados can also be used as grills for cooking hot and fast, but the cone shape of most of them doesn't make them ideal for two-zone cooking. There are a few exceptions, however, including the cookers from Primo, which are oval-shaped. They come with two-position split cooking grates that can be set up high for indirect cooking, or flipped over to position foods down low to the fire for searing. The split, half-moon-shaped grates allow you to accentuate the difference between a direct and an indirect zone by piling charcoal on one side and positioning one grate over it down low for a direct zone, with the other grate up high and away from the fire for an indirect zone.

Cooking Area: 210 square inches (about 10 burgers)

Hitch a Ride: Broil King Keg 5000

Since the heavy ceramic most kamados are made of can crack if dropped or knocked over, they're not the kind of thing you tend to bring to a tailgate. Unless, of course, you have a Broil King Keg. It's made with lightweight fiberglass encased in powder-coated steel, and, while it's not light enough to pick up and carry around, it's easy to lift off the base and pop onto the optional trailer hitch. And if it does get dropped, this baby won't crack like Humpty Dumpty.

Broil King put together a nice package deal for the 5000 that includes a sturdy stand with big wheels and removable side tables, a multifunction tool for handling the grate and removing ash, and a secondary extender rack that hovers above the primary grate to provide extra cook surface. The side tables have handy tool hooks, and there's even a couple of bottle openers built into the handle.

Cooking Area: 280 square inches (about 13 burgers)

Red Is the New Green: Kamado Joe Classic II 18"

The Kamado Joe Classic II 18" is an elegant, well-crafted ceramic cooker that presents strong competition to other 18-inch models in the premium-priced market. This company pays attention to detail and offers upgrades, like top-quality 304 stainless steel cooking grates, as standard features. In 2014, Kamado Joe introduced a unique multilevel grate and heat-deflection system called "Divide and Conquer," which comes standard with this model at no extra charge. The system is a grouping of multilevel racks and deflectors that relieves some of the pain and cost of creating different cooking zones in a round kamado. Kamado Joe is always on the move, innovating and offering unique features not found on other kamados.

Cooking Area: 256 square inches (about 12 burgers)

Kamettle? Kettlelado? The New Weber Summit Charcoal Grill

The Weber Summit Charcoal Grill is a radical departure from George Stephen's original Weber Kettle. It's Weber's first major upgrade to the Kettle in decades. Sure, the prices are in line with Summit gas grills and premium-quality kamados on carts, but they're a big leap up from the Kettles we know and love. It's true that a regular classic Weber Kettle can grill and smoke, but the new Summits are just plain bigger and better in every way. You get more capacity, ease of use, and more versatility. It actually is an excellent dedicated charcoal smoker by design, and the adjustable coal grate that burns directly under the cook surface for better searing also makes the Summit an even better grill than the classic Weber Kettles.

Cooking Area: 452 square inches (about 22 burgers)

BBQ Guru: Homdoor Charcoal Tandoor

The Homdoor Charcoal Tandoor is a traditional Indian clay oven with a stainless steel outer shell. It has no cooking grate. Put meat or vegetables (sweet peppers are especially good) on skewers, saving an onion or potato chunk for last to keep the meat from sliding off into the red-hot coals; lower the skewers into the open, upright cylindrical oven; and you can get tender, juicy seared meat and veggies in four to eight minutes.

Cooking Area: 144 square inches (about 7 burgers)

Big, Bad, and Beautiful: Komodo Kamado Big Bad 32

Komodo Kamado makes some of the highest-quality, most striking cookers we've seen. Stunning assortments of inlaid tile finishes are available, but these cookers aren't just another pretty face. Attention to detail is evident in everything you see and touch, from the 304 stainless steel grates and hinges to the heavy-duty casters. And the casters have to be powerful to support this bad boy—it comes fully assembled and weighs in at almost half a ton. At 32 inches wide, this is the biggest kamado on the market. Want to make it even fancier? Plenty of options are available, including teakwood carts and gas ignition.

Cooking Area: 576 square inches (about 28 burgers)

KAMADO GRILL RECIPES

The following recipes are kamado grill-friendly while also being a treat to the taste buds. Try some of these kamado grill recipes today.

Carolina Style Shrimp

Prepartion time

50 minutes

Ingredients

• 2 half-size disposable aluminum pans

• Vision Grills Carolina Style Dry Rub

- Vision Grills Carolina Style BBQ Sauce

- 2 lbs. of thawed and deveined shrimp

- 1/2 lemon

- 2 sticks salted butter

Instructions

1. Heat your Vision Grill up to 250ºF

2. Pour 2 lbs. of shrimp into one pan

3. Pour enough Vision Grills Carolina BBQ Sauce to coat the bottom of the second pan

4. Pour a generous coating of Vision Grills Carolina Style Dry Rub onto the shrimp

5. Hand toss the shrimp to evenly coat in the rub, add more seasoning if needed

6. Move over the shrimp into the BBQ coated pan

7. Squeeze a half of a lemon onto the shrimp

8. Place two sticks of unsalted butter on top of the shrimp

9. Place the pan of shrimp directly onto your grill rack

10. Close your grill and cook the shrimp for about 35 minutes or until fully cooked to at least 120ºF

11. Remove the pan from the grill with caution and enjoy!

Grilled Coconut Curry Shrimp with

Apricot Dipping Sauce

Prepartion time

1 hour 20 minutes

Ingredients:

- 2 pound 6-8 count shrimp (large shrimp) – peeled and deveined

- ½ cup cream of coconut

- 2 Tbsp. curry powder

- 7 oz. bag shredded coconut

- Cooking oil spray

Apricot Dipping Sauce Ingredients:

- 1 cup apricot preserves

- 1/8 cup rice vinegar

- 1/8 cup Croix Valley Honey Dijon Barbecue 'N Brat Sauce

- 1 Tbsp. red pepper flakes

Instructions

1. Combine cream of coconut and curry powder in a bowl or plastic baggie. Add shrimp. Place in refrigerator for 30 minutes.

2. Put shredded coconut in food processor and chop until fine.

3. Combine Apricot Dipping Sauce ingredients completely, cover and place in refrigerator.

4. After 30 minutes have passed, remove shrimp from coconut curry marinade, cover completely with finely chopped coconut, and lightly spray with cooking oil.

5. Place shrimp on a 375⁰ grill for 8-10 minutes, or until fully cooked and coconut is beginning to brown.

6. Serve shrimp immediately with Apricot Dipping Sauce.

Southern Style Meatloaf

Prepartion time

2 hours 30 minutes

Ingredients:

- 2 lbs Ground Beef

- 1 Onion, minced

- 1 Green Pepper, minced

- 1 Egg

- 2/3 cup Vision Grills BBQ Sauce (Kansas City Style Recommended)

- 3 tbsp Vision Grills BBQ Rub (Kansas City Style Recommended)

- 1/2 cup Italian Bread Crumbs

- 1 tsp Salt

- 1/2 tsp Black Pepper

- 1/2 tsp Garlic Salt

- 1/4 tsp Cayenne Pepper

- 1 tbsp Worcestershire Sauce

- 1 tbsp Hot Sauce

- 1/4 tsp Oregano

- 1/4 tsp Basil

- 1/3 cup 2% Milk

- Meatloaf Done

Instructions

1. In a large bowl, add the Ground Beef, Onion, Pepper, Garlic, Egg, 1/3 cup BBQ Sauce, Italian Bread Crumbs, Salt, Pepper, Cayenne, Basil, Oregano, and Milk

2. Using your hands, knead the meat mixture until everything is well combined

3. Mold the meat into a loaf shape and sprinkle the top with BBQ Rub

4. Start up your Vision Kamado and get it to 350ºF.

5. Place meatloaf in Vision Kamado once it reaches 350ºF

6. Brush with 1/3 cup of BBQ Sauce after the meatloaf reaches 140ºF (about an hour and a half in)

7. Remove when the internal temperature is at 160ºF (about two hours)

Grilled Chicken Quesadilla Sandwich

Prepartion time

20 minutes

Ingredients:

- 4 Chicken Breasts

- 1 package Taco Seasoning

- 1 Green Bell Pepper

- 1 Red Bell Pepper

- 1 Red Onion

- 2 cups Monterey Jack Cheese

- 4 Ciabatta Buns (sliced in half)

- ½ cup Margarine

- 1 Tbsp. Croix Valley Garlic Barbecue Booster

- 1 cup Sour Cream

- 2 Tbsp. Chipotle in Adobo Sauce

- 1 cup Ajvar Relish (Eastern European relish of garlic, peppers and eggplant)

- 1 Tbsp. Olive Oil

- ¼ head Iceberg Lettuce, shredded

- 1 medium Tomato, diced.

Instructions

1.   Lightly oil chicken breasts and coast generously with Taco Seasoning.

2. Grill chicken over medium grill (about 350°F) until internal temperature reaches 165°F.   Let rest 5 minutes then slice into strips.

3. Julienne peppers and onion. Fry in oil until vegetables start to brown. Cover and set aside.

4. Make 4 piles of chicken (as flat as possible) on baking sheet. Top with fried vegetables, ½ cup of cheese, a dash of taco seasoning. Transfer to covered grill and cook until cheese begin to brown.

5. Combine margarine and garlic seasoning. Blend well.

6. Spread margarine garlic mixture on inside of ciabatta buns. Grill until they start to brown.

7. Combine sour cream and chipotle in adobo sauce. Blend well.

8. Spread Ajvar relish on inside of bottom bun.

9. Place chicken/vegetable/cheese stacks on top of Ajvar relish.

10. Top with shredded lettuce and diced tomato..

11. Spread chipotle mixture on inside of top bun and top off sandwich.

12. Serve and enjoy!

Smoked Turkey

Prepartion time

Ingredients:

- 16 – 20-pound thawed turkey

- 3 Garlic Heads

- 6 Vidalia Onions (i.e. Yellow Onions)

- 2 Red Apples

- 4 tablespoons Unsalted Butter

- 1 ⅓ Cups Kosher Salt

- ¼ Cup Whole Peppercorns

- 2 tablespoons Ground black pepper

- 1 tablespoon Onion Powder

- 2 tablespoon Garlic Powder

- 1 ½ tablespoons Garlic Salt

- 1 tablespoon Old Hickory Seasoning

- 2 ½ tablespoons Smoked Paprika

- 11 ¼ cups of Apple Juice (1.5 bottles)

- 1 cup White Vinegar

- 1 ¾ cups White Wine (Something Dry — Like Chardonnay)

- ¾ cups Honey

- ⅓ Cup Vegetable Oil

Supplies:

- 1 Small spool Butcher's Twine

- 4 Wing Pins

- 1 Baster

- 1 Brining Bag, stockpot or bucket (large enough for whole turkey)

- 1 Aluminum Cooking Tray

- *3 Handfuls – Wood Chips or chunks water

soaked for 12 hours

Instructions

The Brine:

1. Dissolve kosher salt in 4 quarts of boiling
water. Then, add to your bucket or stockpot.
Add 7 ½ cups (1 bottle) of apple juice along with
1 ¾ cups White Wine to bucket, bag or stockpot.
Add one head or jar of minced garlic cloves.
Chunk the 3 onions into fourths and add to the
brine. Add ¼ cup of whole black peppercorns.
Place the clean thawed turkey (BREAST SIDE
DOWN) into the brine. Cover the pot (or bucket)
and place in the refrigerator for 12+ hours.

2. *Soak wood chips in separate container of water then set aside for 12 hours while turkey is in the brine. After the 12 hours are up, remove the turkey from the fridge and dry it (thoroughly) with paper towels. Once dry, rub it down with a liberal amount of butter, covering the entire turkey.

Seasoning:

1. Mix Seasonings together into a bowl (1 tablespoon Ground black pepper, 2 tablespoons salt, 2 tablespoons garlic powder, 1 tablespoon garlic salt, 2 tablespoons hickory seasoning)

2. Generously cover turkey with seasonings:

3. Then place the turkey in the aluminum pan (the previously mentioned tin pan).

Cavity Filling:

1. Stuff it with a 3 onions (quartered), 6 cloves garlic, and 2 apples (quartered and cored)

2. Once Stuffed, tie turkey legs together with Butcher's Twine (so the inner contents don't spill out) and secure the wings to the turkey with the pins.

Prep Grill:

1. Heat the grill to 250°-275° and place the lava stone in the brackets.

NOTE:

1. The grill will cool significantly once you place the bird on the grill, so this temp will drop quite a bit. The temp you want to maintain is 225°

2. Before putting the turkey on the grill, sprinkle in wood chips and allow them to char before cooking.

Start Cook:

1. Once the grill is up to temp, place the turkey (still in the pan) on the top grate rack and close the lid.

2. Leave for 1 hour.

Baste:

1. Mix together 3 ¾ cups (1/2 bottle) of apple juice, ¾ cup of honey, and 1 ¾ cup of white vinegar along with ½ tablespoon of garlic salt. Baste the turkey after cooking for 1 hour. Repeat the basting every 2-3 hours for 12-13 hours.

2.   In that time, make sure the temperature does NOT exceed 220°-225°.

NOTE:

1. The meat will need to cook for roughly 30-40 minutes per pound.

Removal:

1. After 12-13 hours, make sure the internal temperature of the thigh registers 165° and the breast registers 155°.

2. Let the turkey rest for 45 minutes.

3. After the allotted resting, it's time to dig in and watch everyone's reaction to this epic meal.

Backyard Turkey

Prepartion time

Ingredients:

• Whole Turkey, 12-14 pounds

• Cold Water, 2 gals (or enough to cover turkey completely)

• Kosher Salt, 1½ cups for each gallon of water

• Clarified Butter, 8 ounces

• Granulated Sugar, 1½ tablespoons

Supplies:

• Food-safe bag or container (look for the food safe symbol – a wine glass and fork)

• Drip Pan (if you want to catch drippings to make turkey gravy)

- Wood Chunks (pecan, apple, cherry, alder, etc.) if smokier flavor is desired

- Turkey Rack (optional, though hot turkeys are easier to remove from the grill on a rack)

- Thermometer (preferably a digital dual-probe smoking thermometer)

- Aluminum Foil

- homemade-smoked-backyard-turkey-kamado-grill-

Instructions

The Brine

1. There is plenty of controversy over whether or not a turkey (or poultry in general) should be brined. We prefer the flavor and juiciness of

brined meat, but encourage you to research the topic and come to your own conclusion.

2. To brine, place the thawed turkey into a food-safe container and completely submerge with water. Add 1½ cups Kosher salt for each gallon of water used. Refrigerate for 12-24 hours, then rinse well and pat completely dry with paper towels.

Tips:

1. Completely thaw turkey before brining (allow approximately 1 day in refrigerator for every 3 pounds of meat that needs to be thawed).

2. Remove the bag of giblets included with the turkey before brining. Look for it in the neck cavity.

3. Don't brine a turkey that has already been brined. Over-brining can dry out the meat and cause it to taste very salty.

4. Feel free to add herbs and spices to brine solution. Oregano, sage, bay leaves, and thyme all go well with turkey.

5. We recommend kosher salt as it dissolves more easily than table salt. If you choose to use table salt, however, cut the salting rate by half.

The Cook

1. Place your lava stone in the Kamado and heat the grill to 275oF. Place a drip pan underneath the turkey rack if you intend to collect the drippings for gravy, otherwise, the lava stone will keep the drippings from causing flare-ups.

Before placing the turkey on the grill, coat it thoroughly with clarified butter.

2. Clarified butter will give you that classic golden brown turkey and is simple to make at home. Simmer ½ pound of unsalted butter until most of the water has boiled off (it will stop bubbling after 30-45 minutes), shut off the heat, skim the milk solids from the top, then ladle out the clear butter remaining.

3. Insert one temperature probe into the thickest part of the turkey breast and set the other to measure the ambient temperature of the grill. Once the breast meat has reached 145oF, add the granulated sugar to the remaining clarified butter and heat up. Brush the sugary butter all over the turkey and let the breast meat reach its

final temperature (165oF). Check the thickest part of the leg meat and make sure it's 175oF. Once final temperatures are met, cover the turkey with foil and let rest for 30-45 minutes. Carve and Enjoy!

Smoked Brisket

Prepartion time

1 hour 40 minutes

Ingredients:

- 8 lb. brisket

Dry rub ingredients:

- 1 Tablespoon kosher salt

- 2 Tablespoons chili powder

- 2 Tablespoons brown sugar

- 1 Teaspoon cumin

- 1 Teaspoon cayenne pepper

- 2 Tablespoons red pepper flakes

- 1 Teaspoon minced dried onion

- 2 Tablespoons paprika

- 2 Tablespoons black pepper

Mop ingredients:

- 1 Can beer

- 1 Cup apple cider vinegar

- 1 Teaspoon kosher salt

- 1 Tablespoon brown sugar

- 2-3 Cloves minced garlic

- 1 Tablespoon red pepper flakes

Other supplies:

- 2 large foil drip pans

- 1-2 large pieces of wood of your choice for smoking the brisket (oak is often a favorite. Aim for 3 inch diameter, 4 inch long pieces if possible)

• Heavy aluminum foil

Instructions

1. Mix ingredients for dry rub together in a medium sized bowl. Set aside.

2. Remove brisket from refrigerator. Rub with yellow mustard and Worcestershire sauce. Coat with dry rub. Let brisket sit and come to room temperature with the rub applied.

3. While the brisket sits, mix your mop ingredients in a large foil drip pan and set aside.

4. Start your Vision Grill and bring it to 225-250 degrees. Throw in a chunk or two of wood of

your choice for smoke and place brisket on grill. Place a foil drip pan under brisket to catch drippings from mop.

5. After the brisket has cooked for an hour, apply a mop every 45 minutes to an hour until the brisket has reached an internal temperature of 190 degrees. Remove from grill and double wrap in heavy aluminum foil. Wrap foil covered brisket in a towel, place in a cooler, and let rest for 1 – 1 1/2 hours. Serve and enjoy!

Campsite Grilled Salmon

Prepartion time

1 hour 30 minutes

Ingredients

- 1 pound salmon filets or steaks ¾ – 1 inch thick (wild caught preferred)

- 2 tablespoons soy sauce

- 2 tablespoons dry sherry

- 1 tablespoon brown sugar

- 1 tablespoon minced fresh ginger root or 1 teaspoon dry ginger

- 2 cloves garlic, minced

- 1 green onion (scallion preferred) thinly sliced

Instructions

1. Rinse fish with cold water and pat dry with paper towels.

2. In zip-lock bag, combine soy sauce, sherry, brown sugar, ginger, and garlic. Add salmon, seal bag, and turn to coat. Refrigerate 30 minutes to 1 hour.

3. Prepare Kamado for baking (set to 275°-350°F). Use Vision Grills lava stone (or pizza stone) on top of cooking grate.

4. Add 2-3 mesquite or hickory wood chunks or 2 handfuls of chips over the charcoal for smoking, close lid until ready to add fish.

5. Place fish on oiled lava or pizza stone skin side down. Grill salmon about 7-10 minutes until fish flakes easily with fork.

6. Carefully remove salmon to serving platter and garnish with green onions.

Smoked Chicken

Prepartion time

5 hours 40 minutes

Ingredients

- 3-5 chicken pieces or whole chicken, rinsed and patted dry with paper towels

- 1 tablespoon packed brown sugar

- 1 ½ tablespoons fresh ground sea salt

- 1 tablespoon of Sriracha™ hot sauce

- ½ teaspoon freshly ground black pepper

Instructions

1. Prepare Kamado for smoking (set to 200° – 250° F) – allow 20-30 minutes.

2. In small bowl combine sugar, salt, and pepper. Coat the chicken evenly with the mixture, place in large zip lock bag and refrigerate for at least 2 hours as long as 6 hours.

3. Add 3-5 mesquite or hickory wood chunks or 2-3 handfuls of chips over the charcoal for smoking, set lava stone on heat hanger bracket, and close lid until ready to add meat.

4. Place chicken skin side down on top grill surface or if using a whole chicken, place belly down or use the Vision Grills roaster.

5. Slow cook 1 ½ to 2 ½ hours until thermometer inserted in thickest parts reads

160-165 ° for a breast and 170-175° for a thigh/leg. Breast will be finished grilling before thighs and legs.

6. Remove from grill, cover with foil, and allow to sit 5-10 minutes before serving.

"St. Louis Style" Babyback Ribs

Prepartion time

5 hours 40 minutes

Ingredients

- 2 pounds trimmed pork loin ribs

- 3-4 tablespoons garlic salt

- ½ teaspoon ground celery seeds

- 2 tablespoons paprika

- 1 tablespoon onion salt

- 2 teaspoons of Ass Kicking™ Wasabi Horseradish Hot sauce or Tabasco™ Chipotle Pepper Sauce

- 1 teaspoon sage

- ½ teaspoon cayenne pepper

- 1 cup apple juice

Instructions

1. In small bowl combine garlic salt, paprika, onion salt, sage, celery seeds and cayenne

pepper in bowl. Sprinkle and rub in mixture on both sides of ribs. Refrigerate for 2+ hours... Or if not don't worry it will still work!

2. Prepare Kamado for grilling (set to 175-200° F) – allow 20-30 minutes. Use a rib rack, Vision Grills lava stone, and heat deflector bracket.

3. Trim excess fat from ribs and remove membrane from back of each rack.

4. Add 3-5 mesquite or hickory wood chunks or 2-3 handfuls of chips over the charcoal for smoking and close lid until ready to add meat.

5. In another small bowl, mix together the hot sauce with apple juice.

6. Place ribs on grill. Cook with lid down for 4-5 hours. Baste with apple juice-hot sauce mixture every hour.

Tokyo Teriyaki Chicken

Prepartion time

6 hours

Ingredients

- 3-4 pounds chicken breast halves, skin on, rinsed in cold water and patted dry

- ¾ cup soy sauce

- 1 teaspoon grated fresh ginger root

- 2 cloves of garlic, crushed

- 1½ teaspoons of Coahuila sauce

- ¼ cup white wine or sherry

- ½ teaspoons of freshly ground sea salt

Instructions

1. Prepare Kamado for grilling (set to 350° F) — allow 20-30 minutes. Use lava stone and heat deflector bracket.

2. Mix soy sauce, ginger, garlic, Coahuila sauce, wine/sherry, and salt in large bowl. Add chicken and marinate 2-6 hours.

3. Place chicken breasts on lower grill surface, skin side down, over medium heat 350° F.

4. Grill breasts turning once after 4-6 minutes. Grill 4-6 minutes longer until chicken is opaque

throughout and the juices run clear or meat thermometer in the thickest portion of breast reads 175-180° F.

5. Remove and cover with foil. Allow to sit 10 minutes before serving.

Sizzling Diablo Shrimp

Prepartion time

40 minutes

Ingredients

• ½ cup butter

• 4 garlic cloves, minced

• 1 teaspoon cayenne pepper

- 1 teaspoon cumin

- ½ cup white wine

- 4 tablespoons flat leaf parsley, chopped

- 1-1 ½ pounds shrimp, peeled and deveined, tail on

- ½ teaspoon coarse salt

- ¼ teaspoon of fresh ground pink peppercorn pepper

Instructions

1. Preheat Kamado to 400°F with Vision Grills lava stone (or pizza stone) – allow 20 minutes.

2. Melt butter in small saucepan over medium/low heat. Add garlic, cumin, and

cayenne pepper. Cook until garlic is soft. Be careful not to burn the garlic. Add wine, raise heat to med/high and cook until reduced by half and allow to cool for 10-15 minutes. Stir in 2 Tbsp. parsley.

3. Pour butter mixture over shrimp in bowl. Add salt and toss shrimp to coat.

4. Grill Shrimp over high heat for 3-4 minutes on grill stone, turning once after 1½ – 2 minutes.

5. Remove from grill and enjoy.

Bacon Wrapped Tenderloins

Prepartion time

50 minutes

Ingredients

- 2 (1.5 lbs.) pork tenderloins, trimmed of fat and silver skin removed

- 3 tablespoons Dijon-style mustard

- 1 ½ tablespoons green peppercorns (packed in water) drained

- 3 tablespoons coarsely ground 5 peppercorn blends (equal parts black, green, pink, & white peppercorns, and whole allspice in a peppermill or grinder)

- 8 fresh large sage leaves

- 8-10 slices bacon

- ½ teaspoons of freshly ground sea salt sprinkled over filleted meat

- 10 inch bamboo skewers (soak 20-30 in water) or metal works wiped with olive oil

Instructions

1. Prepare Kamado for grilling (set to 450 – 550° F). Use Vision Grills lava stone (or pizza stone) on top of cooking grate and allow 20-30 minutes.

2. Using a sharp knife, make a cut lengthwise down the center of the tenderloin through two-thirds of the thickness, spread meat open, and flatten slightly.

3. Spread mustard in a thin layer over the tenderloin. Scatter the green peppercorns evenly over the opened meat & press lightly with your hands. Sprinkle 1 tablespoon of the peppercorn blend evenly over the opened meat. Place sage leaves in a row down the center.

4. Shape the tenderloin back to its original shape. Wrap bacon slices around tenderloin and use bamboo skewers to secure bacon on the tenderloin.

5. Place the tenderloins on the hottest part of the grill and cook, turning occasionally, until well

browned on all sides (approximately 10 minutes). Move tenderloins to upper grill surface and continue to cook, turning occasionally, until thermometer inserted into the center registers 145° F. Remove the tenderloins from the grill and allow to sit, loosely covered with foil, for 5-10 minutes before serving.

6. Slice the tenderloins on the diagonal.

Bacon/Chicken Kabobs

Prepartion time

50 minutes

INGREDIENTS:

- 1 package chicken tenders

- 1 package thin-sliced bacon

- Your favorite BBQ seasoning

- Your favorite BBQ sauce

- Wooden or metal BBQ skewers

Instructions

1. Before you begin assembling the kabobs, heat your grill. Use a diffuser and place a drip pan on the bottom shelf. Cooking with bacon will cause flare ups if you don't' catch the grease!! Heat grill to about 400 degrees.

2. Cut the chicken tenders into one inch pieces. Take a slice of bacon and thread about an inch from the end onto the skewer. Then, add a piece

of chicken, weave the bacon around the chicken and run skewer through it again. Repeat until bacon is gone. You should get 4-5 pieces of chicken on each skewer. Gently pull the chicken and pack up the skewer so that it's not all mashed together.

3. Sprinkle both sides with BBQ rub. Place the kabobs on the top rack of the hot grill. Turn them over after 15-20 minutes. You can see the chicken is partially cooked and bacon is beginning to brown in spots. Continue cooking until chicken and bacon is done. They should be done in approximately 25 minutes. If grill is a little hotter or cooler, grilling time could vary.

4. Once done, remove from grill and lightly brush with your favorite BBQ sauce. Enjoy.

Miso Marinated Mushrooms

Prepartion time

30 minutes

Ingredients:-

• 20 closed cup or button mushrooms

• 2 tablespoons brown miso paste

• 2 tablespoons lemon juice

• 2 tablespoons brown sugar

• 1 tablespoon soy sauce (or Tamari)

Instructions

1. Take a glass bowl and add all the ingredients except the mushrooms and use a fork or whisk to blend to an even consistency. This will take you about 5 minutes at most.

2. Set your grill up for indirect cooking. You can roast miso marinated mushrooms at pretty much any temperature between 120 - 180°C (250 - 350°F) which makes them supremely versatile and easy to fit in with other food that you are cooking at the same time - clearly the higher the temperature the quicker they cook. I like to do mine at about 150°C for 20 minutes or so.

3. Just hold the mushroom by the stalk and dunk it in the miso marinade and place it on the grill. Close the lid and let them cook.

4. The ones that you see on my Monolith above are fresh on the grill so they still look full of moisture. As they cook, so that moisture will be released and the mushrooms will darken in colour and become flaccid.

5. If you look carefully you'll be able to see the heat deflector (half) stone is over the fire so that my miso marinated mushrooms are cooking indirectly while the avocado and bacon skewers and leeks are cooking directly over the coals.

6. Because there's sugar in the marinade you may find that they stick to the grill grate a little so just ease them with a spatula when it's time to serve. In fact the point at which the marinade gets sticky and the mushrooms get soft and

wrinkly is actually a good sign that the mushrooms are cooked.

7. I keep service very simple, just on a tray with a cocktail stick. Serve immediately as they're much better when warm.

Plancha Grilled Mini Lamb Koftas With Yoghurt Raita Dip

Prepartion time

35 minutes

Ingredients:-

• 500g ground lamb

- 1 small red onion, very finely chopped or minced

- 10g (1/3 cup) chopped fresh flat leaf parsley

- 10g (1/3 cup) chopped fresh mint

- 1 teaspoon ground cumin

- 1 teaspoon ground coriander

- 1 fresh chilli finely chopped

- 1 beaten egg

- 1 garlic clove, crushed

- 1 teaspoon of cracked black pepper

- ½ teaspoon salt

- 1 tablespoon olive oil

Instructions

1. Making the mini lamb koftas couldn't be easier. Just get a large mixing bowl, throw all the ingredients (except the olive oil) into the bowl and get your hands in to give it a thorough mix.

2. Next form the koftas by taking a small amount of the meat mix and forming it into a ball that's about 1cm (½ inch) in diameter.

3. To cook, I used the plancha over gentle direct heat. Interestingly I found it useful to place the plancha on a Monolith wok stand because this gave me a high heat central area of the plancha with the cooler peripheral area. This made it easier to ensure that the mini lamb koftas were

cooked all the way through without the outside getting burnt.

4. If you don't have a wok stand to hand then the trick is to use a splash of the olive oil, gentle heat and keep the koftas moving with a spatula.

5. After about 15 minutes use an instant read thermometer to check that the internal temperature of the kofta has reached 75°C (165°F)

Serving Mini Lamb Koftas

1. Use a large plate and place a bowl of raita in the centre.

2. Spear every lamb kofta with a cocktail stick and place them on the plate surrounding the

bowl of raita. You guests can then take a stick, dunk their kofta in the raita and then savour the flavour.

Deep Fried Mozzarella Balls With Spicy Dipping Sauce

Prepartion time

30 minutes

Ingredients:-

For the deep fried mozzarella balls

• 1 mozzarella 400g block

• 3 tablespoons plain flour (well seasoned with salt and pepper)

- 2 beaten eggs

- 100g panko breadcrumbs

- 1 teaspoon garlic salt

- 1 teaspoon dried oregano

- vegetable oil for deep-frying

- For the dipping sauce

- 1 x 400g carton of passata

- 1 clove of garlic (chopped)

- ½ teaspoon chilli flakes

- 1 teaspoon granulated sugar

- 1 tablespoon olive oil

Instructions

1. Cut the mozzarella block into 1cm cubes and then leave them to sit on kitchen paper for 10 minutes.

2. Put the flour, egg and panko breadcrumbs into separate bowls and line them up in the order described. Add the garlic salt and oregano into the breadcrumbs and get your hands in a toss the mix.

3. Line a baking tray with baking parchment and place it next to the panko breadcrumbs - this will be the tray where you place the finish mozarella balls.

4. Dip each cube of mozzarella first in the flour, then the beaten egg and finally the panko breadcrumbs. As you complete the coating, line

them up on the parchment lined tray and then place them in the freezer for 20 minutes.

5. To make the sauce, heat the olive oil, add the garlic and gently cook until really soft. Add the chilli flakes, passata and sugar, and simmer for 15 minutes until thickened. The sauce will be pretty smooth but you can give it a whizz with a stick blender if you wish.

6. Add the vegetable oil to the wok until it is no more than a third full, place it over the charcoal heat and monitor the temperature reaches 150°C. Take the mozzarella balls from the freezer and fry them in batches of half a dozen until golden brown, remove with a slotted spoon and drain on kitchen paper. Spear each deep

fried mozzarella ball with a cocktail stick and serve immediately with the warm dipping sauce.

Vegan Mini Sausage Rolls Recipe

Prepartion time

1 hour

Ingredients:-

* 2 sticks (approx 1 cup) of celery, finely chopped

* 1 onion (approx 1 cup) finely chopped

* 1 tablespoon olive oil

* 500 g chestnut mushrooms

- 2 cloves of garlic finely chopped

- 1 tablespoon wholegrain mustard

- 1 tablespoon dark soy sauce

- 100 ml white wine

- sea salt

- freshly ground black pepper

- 80 g fresh white breadcrumbs

- ½ bunch of fresh flat-leaf parsley

- 1 teaspoon finely chopped thyme leaves

- 2 sheets of vegan ready-rolled puff pastry = 640g (I used Jus Rol)

- almond milk

- 2 teaspoons sesame seeds

Instructions

1. The first job is to prepare the filling which I have done in the frying pan over direct heat. Alternatively you could use the wok and wok stand.

2. Peel and finely chop the onion, then trim and finely chop the celery.

3. Heat 1 tablespoon of olive oil in your pan / wok and add the chopped veg. Cook for 10 to 15 minutes, or until golden.

4. Meanwhile, finely chop the mushrooms. I take the stalks out first because that makes the mushrooms easier to chop and then I chop the stalks separately. Peel and crush in the garlic,

then add the chopped mushrooms and garlic to the pan.

Vegan sausage stuffing

1. Cook for a further 5 minutes, or until the mushrooms start to soften.

2. Next add the mustard, wine and soy sauce, season with salt and pepper, cook for 5 to 10 minutes, or until all the liquid has boiled and bubbled away. Set aside to cool.

3. Turn out the cooled mushroom mixture into a large mixing bowl and add the breadcrumbs. Finely chop and add the parsley leaves and thyme leaves.

4. Stir well to combine everything together and adjust seasoning to taste.

5. Now set up your barbecue for indirect cooking at 200°C (395°F). For my Monolith kamado this means having the heat deflector stones in situ.

6. Cut the sheets of puff pastry in half lengthways so you have four equal-sized pieces.

Stuffing the Puff Pastry

1. Spoon a quarter of the mushroom mixture along the middle of one length of pastry, moulding it into a long sausage shape with the back of a spoon.

2. Brush the almond milk along the pastry edges, then carefully fold one of the long sides of the pastry up over the filling.

3. Press the edges to seal, then crimp with a fork. Repeat with the remaining ingredients until you have four long rolls, then cut each length to create your vegan mini sausage rolls.

4. Place the mini rolls closely together on the pizza stone (this helps keep the ends moist), brush with the almond milk and sprinkle over the sesame seeds.

5. Place the pizza stone on the 2nd tier grill grate so that you have a good gap between the pizza stone and the heat deflector stones and bake for 20 minutes until the pastry is crisp and golden.

6. I served my vegan mini sausage rolls very simply with a dollop of homemade tomato ketchup.

Cauliflower Pakora Florets With Pomegranate Raita Dip

Prepartion time

50 minutes

Ingredients:-

• 1 teaspoon cumin seeds

• 150ml (10 tablespoons) natural yoghurt

• Seeds from ½ pomegranate

- Salt & pepper to season

- 1 tablespoon vegetable oil

- Note: You can turn this whole recipe vegan by substituting with soy yoghurt.

Method:-

Heat the vegetable oil in a small pan, add the cumin seeds and cook until they start to pop. Pour the yoghurt into your serving bowl, take the cumin seeds off the heat and stir into the yoghurt. Season with salt and pepper, add the pomegranate seeds and stir.

Place the bowl in the refrigerator for an hour or so to give a little time for all the flavours to mingle.

Cauliflower Pakora Florets

Prepartion time

12 minutes

Ingredients

- 1 small cauliflower cut into small florets*

- 200g (1½ cups) gram flour

- 180ml (¾ cup) water, approximately

- 2 teaspoons garam masala

- ½ teaspoon dried chilli flakes

- 2 tablespoons chopped fresh coriander (cilantro)

- Salt and pepper to season

- Vegetable oil for deep frying

Instructions

1. Bring a pan of water to the boil and blanch the cauliflower florets for 2 minutes and drain.

2. In a mixing bowl add the gram flour, spices and season with salt and pepper. Next add enough cold water to make a thick batter.

3. Fill your wok ⅓ full with vegetable oil and heat until you reach a temperature of about 150°C (300°F), dip your cauliflower florets in batter to ensure that they are fully coated, shake off any excess then fry in batches until puffed, crisp and golden.

4. When cooked, drain on paper towel and the serve your cauliflower pakora florets with the raita.

Barbeque Roast Beef – Indirect BBQ Cooking

Prepartion time

4 hours 10 minutes

Ingredients:-

• Beef joint of 1.5kg or 3.3lbs

• Worcestershire sauce (or your favorite bbq marinade)

• Salt and pepper

Instructions

1. Place the beef in a plastic bag and pour in ½ cup (100ml) of your marinade, seal the bag and refrigerate for as long as you have patience! A minimum of two or three hours is ideal and you can enhance the process by injecting marinade. Turn the beef occasionally.

2. When the grill is ready, season the beef well with salt and pepper and cook just as if you were roasting. I like my beef rare so I'll be going for 15 minutes per pound plus 15 minutes at 200°C or 400°F but you may want to do slightly longer depending on your preference. For the size of joint we're using the cooking time should be 65

minutes. Remember that if the outside is well cooked then it's safe to eat.

3. Serve with potatoes in creme fraiche, a green salad and perhaps some Cabernet Sauvignon in a large glass?

Sunblush Tomato And Pesto Puff Pastry Bites

Prepartion time

30 minutes

Ingredients:-

For The Pesto

• 80g (½ cup) pine nuts

- 30ml (2 tablespoons) olive oil

- A 60g handful of basil

- 1 tablespooon lemon juice

- 1 small clove of garlic

- ¼ teaspoon salt

- To Complete The Sunblush Tomato And Pesto Puff Pastry Bites

- 1 sheet of ready rolled vegan puff pastry (I used Jus-Rol)

- 1 jar sunblush tomatoes

- Pesto

Instructions

For The Pesto

1. Toast the pine nuts by gently heating them in a dry frying pan for a couple of minutes.

2. Put all the ingredients into a food processor and blitz

3. Pour off any excess oil floating on top of the pesto. I wouldn't normally do this to a pesto but I found that the oil can very quickly make the puff pastry go soggy and then it doesn't puff up as well when you cook it.

To Assemble The Sunblush Tomato And Pesto Puff Pastry Bites

1. Roll out your sheet of puff pastry and cut it into 2cm (1 inch) squares and lay them out on your pizza stone.

2. Add ½ teaspoon of pesto to each square and top off with a piece of sunblush tomato. You may need to cut up your sunblush tomatoes depending on how big they are.

3. Set up your grill for indirect cooking at 200°C (395°F) - for my Monolith kamado this means having the heat deflrctor stones in place and then I'll be using the 2nd tier grill grate upon which to site my pizza stone.

4. Transfer the pizza stone to the grill and bake your pastries for about 15 minutes until the pastry squares have puffed up and turned a golden brown colour.

5. Serve immediately.

Burger And Fries On The Kamado Grill

Prepartion time

1 hour 40 minutes

Ingredients:-

• Potatoes for fries

• Duck fat (or goose fat)

• Ground beef for burgers

Instructions

1. Cut up your potatoes for fries and throw them into boiling water for 10 minutes, drain thoroughly and dry with a little kitchen paper.

2. Allow the fries to cool, place them in an oven tray and then spoon over the duck fat and leave them to sit for an hour - this allows the fat time to penetrate the potato and really deliver that crisp texture that we are looking for.

3. Next we need a blast of heat.

4. Get your kamado going really hot and set it up for indirect cooking (caution – use heat resistant gloves to insert the heat deflector stones).

5. The fries will cook at 180°C or 350°F in about 30 minutes so when you get to half time, lay the

burgers on the grate above and let them have fifteen minutes.

6. When the fries are ready (again with heat resistant gloves) remove the oven tray and the heat deflector stones and give the burgers 5 minutes grilling on each side to brown them.

7. Drain the fries and transfer them to a warm serving dish, place the burgers on top and the choice of barbecue sauce is up to you.....or why not make your own homemade ketchup?

Kamado BBQ Beef Burger Recipe

Prepartion time

35 minutes

Ingredients:-

• Ground Beef (allow 125g per serving)

• salt 1g per serving ie. 1% of total weight

• freshly ground black pepper (0.5g per serving)

Instructions

1. Place your ground beef in a bowl, mix in the salt and pepper and make the patties.

2. The absolute must from a food hygiene perspective is that a burger should be cooked through and the technical capability of a kamado makes it just that little bit easier.

3. If you have a two zone oval kamado then set it up with one heat deflector stone so that you

can cook both directly and indirectly as shown below.

4. Otherwise set yourself up for indirect cooking at a temperature of approx 120 - 140°C or 250 - 275°F, place your patties on the cooking grate over a drip tray, close the lid and cook for 15 minutes.

5. This will ensure that your burger is cooked through but you'll notice that it's not crisp and caramelized on the outside and that's because the Maillard reaction doesn't take place until you are over 150°C (300°F). (It's the Maillard reaction that browns, caramelizes, crisps and therefore adds flavour).

6. So to get that brown, crispy and tasty result that we're looking for it's now time to cook

directly for 5 minutes on each side. With your oval kamado it's easy, just move the burgers over to the other side of your kamado otherwise get your heat resistant gloves on, remove the heat deflector stone and set up for direct grilling.

7. Get your kamado to 250°C or 480°F and replace the patties on the grill. Close the lid and then flip after 5 minutes. Take care when opening the lid at these temperatures, lift the lid gently so that you don't get a rush of oxygen into the fire and flare up.

8. Once flipped, close the lid again, shut the top vent and bottom damper and continue to cook for another 5 minutes. There you have it, the perfect kamado bbq beef burger recipe, so much better than simply grilling.

Rotisserie Chicken And Mushroom Recipe

Prepartion time

1 hour 50 minutes

Ingredients:-

- 12 large skinless boneless chicken thighs

- 13 large field mushrooms

- For the rotisserie chicken and mushroom marinade

- 120ml or ½ cup vegetable oil

- 3 cloves garlic crushed

- 1 fresh red chilli finely chopped

- Juice and zest of 1 lemon

- ½ tablespoon freshly chopped rosemary

- ½ tablespoon freshly chopped thyme

- ½ teaspoon salt

Instructions

1. Place all the ingredients for the marinade into a bowl, add the chicken and work the marinade around so that it gets to contact all the chicken. Allow to marinate for 30 minutes, there's no need to refrigerate for this short a time.

2. While that marinade is working it's magic, peel the mushrooms and remove the stalks.

3. When the marinade time is up, start with one mushroom and carefully thread the rotisserie skewer through the centre where the stalk was. Next thread on a chicken thigh (together with a much of the solid part of the marinade as possible) then another mushroom and so on.

4. Hold onto the marinade and use as a mop in the latter stages of cooking.

5. Provided you pierce every layer through the centre then you'll have an evenly balanced skewer.

6. The thirteenth mushroom just helps to keep the structure of the "kebab" and help keep all the chicken supremely moist.

7. Set your grill up at approximately 170 - 180°C (about 340 - 350°F) and you're ready to cook.

8. When done, place your rotisserie chicken and mushroom skewer into position, close the lid on your grill and spit roast for about 45 minutes.

9. When the time is up, stop the rotisserie turning and insert an instant read thermometer into the kebab from one end along the length of the skewer. Take care not to have the probe touching the skewer and this will give you an accurate temperature at the core - it should be a minimum of 70°C (160°F).

10. If close to this temperature then brush on some of the marinade to the surface of your rotisserie chicken and mushroom, set the rotisserie turning and grill for another ten minutes. This will add an extra layer of carmelisation (and flavour) but don't do this too

early otherwise you'll get some bitter specs of burnt garlic on the surface.

11. When you've reached core temperature, remove the spit from the heat and allow to rest for 10 minutes. Slide out the skewer and serve your guests with a chicken thigh on a field mushroom bed.

BBQ Chicken Tikka Kebabs

Prepartion time

2 days

Ingredients:-

• 8 skinless, boneless chicken thighs

- 2 Onions

- 5 cloves garlic

- 250ml or 2 cups natural yogurt

- 3 fresh red chillies

- 2 teaspoons ground ginger

- 2 teaspoons turmeric

- 1 teaspoon cumin

- 1 teaspoon ground coriander

- Juice of 1 lemon

Instructions

1. Pop the peeled onions, garlic and chillies into a food processor and blitz until they form a

rough paste, add the remaining ingredients and mix again thoroughly and the marinade is done.

2. Place the chicken thighs into the marinade, cover with stretch wrap and refrigerate for 24 to 48 hours.

3. When you're ready to cook, remove the chicken thighs from the marinade and pat them dry with kitchen towel. This removes any excess marinade ensuring that the outside of the meat will seal and keep the juices in. (If there's too much marinade on your chicken it'll just go soggy.)

4. Remove the grill plate and get the kamado well cranked up to about 300°C or 600°F and then thread a whole chicken thigh onto an individual skewer, threading it right up to the

handle. Using heat resistant gloves, place the skewer tips in the hot charcoal and rest the skewers vertically on the inside of the kamado.

5. Cook for 10 minutes and you'll have bbq chicken tikka kebabs to die for. Serve up with naan bread and cucumber raita and marvel at the versatility of your kamado ceramic tandoor.

Kamado Baked Croissants

Prepartion time

12 hours

Ingredients:-

• There's gluten in the flour.

For the starter culture

- 2oz or 25g dried yeast

- ½ cup or 120ml warm water

- ½ cup or 120ml warm milk

- ½ cup or 85g plain flour

- 2 tablespoons granulated sugar

For the bread dough

- 3 cups or 335g plain flour

- 2 teaspoons salt

- 12 oz or 340g unsalted butter

In addition

• You will need extra flour to use when rolling out your pastry and a beaten egg to use as an egg wash prior to baking.

Instructions

1. Place all the batter ingredients in a mixing bowl, take a hand whisk and combine until you have a smooth paste. Cover and set this aside for 2 hours so that yeast can feed and multiply – you'll be able to see this happening because the batter will start to bubble and increase in volume.

2. Cut your butter up into ½ " or 1cm cubes and keep it chilled

3. In a separate mixing bowl take half the butter, all the flour, salt and using your hands gently squeeze the flour into the butter just so that everything starts to come together (you're not looking to work the flour completely into the butter). When done, put this bowl in the refrigerator until your batter.

4. When the yeast culture batter is ready, take your flour and butter mix out of the refrigerator and add the batter to it in order to make a nice dough. This dough now needs to be rolled out 4 times over a period of time and at the end of every rolling out, more of the butter is added.

5. Using additional flour to stop the dough from sticking, roll it out. Add a third of the butter cubes, fold it up and return it to the refrigerator

for 15 minutes. Repeat this process for a second and a third time until you have used up the remaining cubes of butter.

6. After the third 15 minutes in the refrigerator, roll the dough out for a fourth time until it's about ¼ inch or 6mm thick then fold it up, wrap it in stretch wrap and return it to the refrigerator overnight.

7. On the morning of the cookout, take your dough out of the refrigerator (if you want to roll it out again then no problem) and cut 16 triangle shapes out of it.

8. Roll the triangles up from base to top and set them out on a lightly greased baking tray with a nice bit of room between them so that they can double their size.

9. Let them sit like this for a couple of hours at room temperature. This gives the croissants time to expand and you time to light the kamado and set it up for indirect cooking.

10. After the 2 hours, brush the croissants with the beaten egg wash and place them in the kamado for 15 – 20 minutes at 400°F or 200°C over indirect heat until golden brown.

11. Serve them straight out of the oven with a pot of freshly brewed coffee.